A tailored education experience —

Sherpath
book-organized
collections

Sherpath is the digital teaching and learning technology designed specifically for healthcare education.

Sherpath book-organized collections offer:

Objective-based, digital lessons, mapped chapter-by-chapter to the textbook, that make it easy to find applicable digital assignment content.

Adaptive quizzing with personalized questions that correlate directly to textbook content.

Teaching materials that align to the text and are organized by chapter for quick and easy access to invaluable class activities and resources.

Elsevier eBooks that provide convenient access to textbook content, even offline.

VISIT
myevolve.us/sherpath today to learn more!

21-CS-0280 TM/AF 6/21

ELSEVIER

T015622O